POSITIVE PARENTING

Peaceful Guilt-Free Strategies for
Discipline and Development of Happy
Confident Children

Marianne Kind

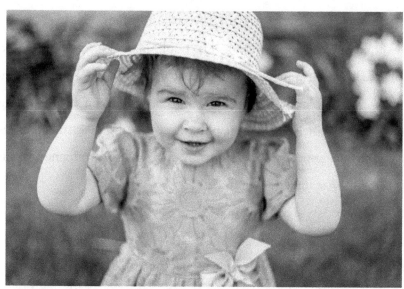

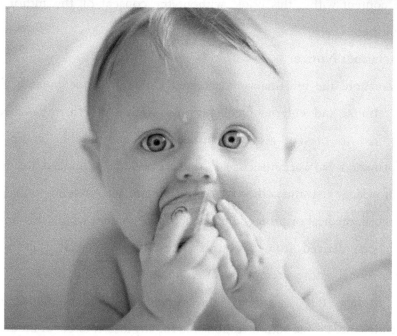

Table Of Contents

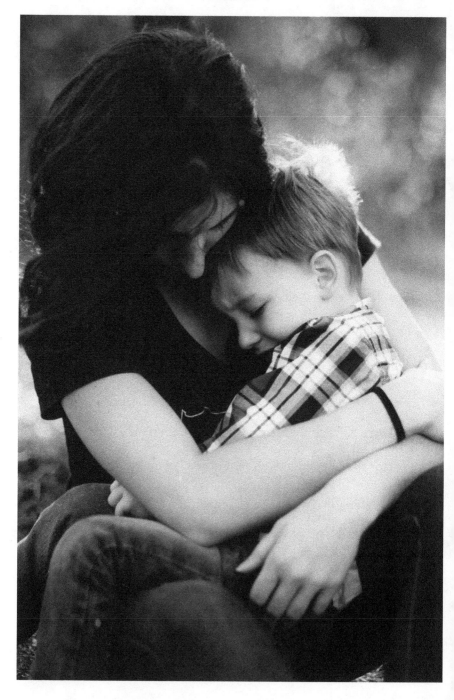

1.

Steps to Becoming a Peaceful Parent

Becoming a peaceful parent is not always an easy task. Modern life demands can mean that parents are already under stress, deadlines, and pressures even before children are thrown into the mix. Some days, it can feel like our kids are testing the limits of our patience to the breaking point.

Depending on the situation, reacting may put a quick stop to misbehavior, but it rarely allows for teaching moments to occur. Reacting leads to yelling, ordering children to their rooms, in-the-moment punishments, and often overlooks or ignores teaching opportunities. It's also stressful for parents! Too much anger can make parenting unenjoyable and leave you feeling out of control.

Even the most practiced of parents will have moments when calm seems far away and anger flares. In the face of these moments, it's all too easy for positive parenting strategies to go out the window.

Patience Is Vital—Tips and Techniques to Stay Calm in Critical Situations.

Let's look at some mindful strategies for staying calm, finding patience, and responding rather than reacting:

Commit Yourself

This is not an instant-fix tip, but it does help. Making a formal commitment to yourself that you are not going to lose your temper won't stop it from happening ever again – but over time, this consciously made commitment can help you to be more aware of what's going on situationally and internally when you lose your temper. The parenting situations that bring them on, you can start to make more mindful choices in those frustrating moments. Don't give up. As you begin to notice your anger and become better at managing it, your parenting's effectiveness can increase. As that increases, your child's misbehavior will start to decrease. Decreased misbehavior means less stress, which leads to less anger. In other words, consistently being mindful of your frustration over time can lead to a happy snowball of more enjoyable parenting!

Could you Put it in Perspective?

It's not uncommon for overstressed parents to start asking questions like, 'Why are they doing this? Is it because I'm not a good parent? Am I failing somehow?' 'What if they NEVER learn? What if they end up living under a bridge?' Try to calm down and remember that button-pushing, boundary testing, and misbehavior are all normal. They are a healthy part of your child's attempts to experiment with and understand the world around her. Expect that these things will happen. Recognize that your job is not to eliminate such issues overnight, but to guide your children through the process of growth and discovery that comes with learning how to function safely and healthily in the human condition. Your child's behavior is outside the norm; seek specific guidance from your pediatrician.

Take a Deep Breath

Believe it or not, taking a moment to breathe is more than just pat advice. A few calming breaths can be done in under thirty seconds but do wonders to calm down. Deep breathing delivers oxygen to your blood and brain, helping you relax and think more clearly under stress. This exercise can also allow you to pause and collect yourself before you react to breathe with you.

Splash Water on Your Face

The face helps some people to change their internal landscape just enough to step away from the anger. However, only apply this strategy or any strategy that requires you to step away.

Add New Tools to Your Toolbox

Come up with a list of anger management techniques that have worked for you in the past, then go out and find some new ones to add to the list (hint: this is a great place to start!). When you feel anger coming on, pull one of these 'tools' from your anger management toolbox—being prepared with options when things can do wonders for one's ability to regain control.

Remember that Feelings are Contagious

If you are angry, anxious, or stressed, your children probably will be too. Kids are smart—even when parents control their reactions, little ones will likely pick up on the fact that mom or dad is upset. This can stress children out and lead to further misbehavior, adding fuel to the fire. Taking a moment to remember that our anger is making things worse can sometimes give us pause; we need to apply a calm-down strategy.

Take a Break

Sometimes taking a short break can give you the space you need to regain your calm. This strategy can even be turned into a teaching moment as you model a healthy coping technique for your child. Tell your children that you are upset, and you need to take a break to calm down. Then leave (providing it is safe to do so), take a quick walk, run through some breathing exercises, do some yoga poses—whatever helps you calm down best. When you return, you can ask your children why they thought you needed a break and jump into a teaching moment around coping with difficult emotions.

How to Stop Yelling at Your Child

A common but unfortunate side effect of anger is yelling. While yelling can sometimes put a stop to misbehavior at the moment, it's less effective in the long run for promoting discipline. It can also undermine parent-child relationships, create stress for everyone involved, and interfere with authentic communication attempts. That being said, it's probably not the end of the world if you yell at your kids one day. Beating yourself up over it is usually not helpful. Just as you want to teach your kids to learn from their mistakes and move on, if you yell at your child, learn from the experience, make amends, forgive yourself, and then move on so that positive parenting can take effect.

Discussing the yelling that is sometimes necessary for safety situations, such as warning your child to get out of the road in the face of an oncoming vehicle. The focus here is on yelling as the result of anger or other negative emotions.

Let's stock up that peaceful parent toolbox a little more by looking at some tips and tricks to stop yelling:

- **Ask your kids to explain their feelings**. It can be accessible in a heated moment to feel like your child is acting out just to make you angry. Understanding the real reasons why a child has misbehaved can help add a little perspective and cool the fuse of our anger.

  It's also suitable for kids who need to be heard and validated at least as much as adults do. Just listening to your child's feelings may be enough to reduce the misbehavior, which will, in turn, help your frustration levels.

- **Get a stress ball**. Many people swear by these small devices. Having a stress ball to squeeze can give you something else to focus on when you're about to lose your cool, and the physical use of your hands can help take the edge off of your stress. You can try keeping one in your bag and pulling it out in heated moments.

- **Don't take it personally**. Know that your child's misbehavior is not personal. Transgression is a normal part of the development and is expected as she learns to self-regulate her actions and emotions. Taking it personally will not only add to your stress at the moment, but it can also lead to resentment over time.

- **Disengage**. Until you can calm your anger, do nothing. If you've already started yelling, stop where you're at. The more often you stop yourself, the more quickly you'll notice that you're crying. Eventually, this strategy can help you avoid yelling altogether.

- **Don't force a teaching moment**. Positive teaching moments can't happen when you're yelling. Wait until you've calmed down before trying to teach your child.

- **Take preventative action**. If you know that having the plant knocked over sets you off, put it out of reach. If you know that your children's' fighting over a particular toy will lead to your yelling, put the toy away until they are ready to play without fighting. If you know that going home from the park will lead to yelling, if your children refuse to come home, make a plan to deal with their refusal more constructively. Identifying situations that lead to yelling can help you eliminate them when appropriate and plan personal coping strategies when not.

- **Set realistic expectations**. Frustration is more likely to occur when your kids fail to meet the behavioral expectations you've set for them. Setting expectations that are too advanced for their developmental level will only lead to 'failures' on their part and frustration for both of you. Give them —and yourself— plenty of opportunities to succeed by setting behavioral expectations that are in keeping with their developmental level.

2.

Temperament and Behavior

Temperament is defined as the heritable and biologically based core that influences the style of approach and response of a person. The child's early temperament traits usually predict their adult temperament.

The child's behavior is the outcome of their temperament and the progress of their emotional, cognitive, and physical development. It is influenced by their beliefs about themselves, about you, and the world in general. While it is inborn and inherent, there are specific ways to help your toddler manage it to their advantage.

Nine dimensions or traits related to temperament:

The activity level pertains to the amount of physical motion that your toddler demonstrates while engaged in some activities. It also includes their inactive periods.

- Is your child a restless spirit that cannot sit still for long and always wants to move around?

- Is your toddler the quiet, the little one enjoys playing alone or watching TV?

14

Rhythmicity refers to predictability or unpredictability of physical and biological functions which include hunger, bowel movement, and sleeping.

- Does your child thrive on routine and follow regular eating or sleeping patterns?

- DO they display unpredictable behavior and dislike routine?

Attention span and persistence are the skills to remain focused on the activity for a certain period.

- Does your toddler stick to complete a task?

- Are they easily frustrated and look for another activity?

Initial Response (Approach or Withdrawal) refers to the reaction to something new and unfamiliar. It describes their initial feelings to a stimulus like a new person, place, toy, and food. Their reaction is shown by their mood or facial expressions like smiling or motor activity, such as reaching for a toy or swallowing food. Negative responses include withdrawal, crying, fussing, pushing away, or spitting the food.

- Are they wary or reluctant around unfamiliar situations or strangers?

- Do they welcome new faces and adjust comfortably with new settings?

The intensity of the reaction is associated with the level of response to any event or situation. Toddlers respond differently to events around them. Some shriek with happiness or giggle joyfully, others throw fits, and many barely react to what is happening.

- Do you always experience trying to guess the reaction of your child over something?

- Does your child explicitly show their emotions?

Adaptability is the child's ability to adjust themself to change over time.

- Is your child capable of adjusting themself to sudden changes in plans or disruptions of their routine?

- Distractibility is the level of the child's willingness to be distracted. It relates to the effects of an outside stimulus on your child's behavior.

- Can your child focus on their activity despite the distraction that surrounds him?

- Are they unable to concentrate when people or other activities are going on in the environment?

Quality of mood is related to how your child sees the world in their own eyes and understanding. Some react with acceptance and pleasure while other children scowl with displeasure just "because" they feel like it.

- Do they display mood changes always?

- Do they generally have a happy disposition?

Sensory Threshold is linked to sensitivity to sensory stimulation. Children sensitive to stimulation require a careful and gradual introduction to new people, experiences, or objects.

- Is your child easily bothered by bright lights, loud sounds, or food textures?

- Are they totally undisturbed with such things and welcome them as such?

There are three main types of toddlers:

- Active or Feisty Toddlers—These children have a tremendous amount of energy, which they show even while inside their mothers' uterus, like lots of moving and kicking. As an infant, they move around, squirm, and crawl all over the place. As toddlers, they climb, run, jump, and even fidget a lot to release their energy. They become excited while doing things or anxious around strangers or new situations.

They are naturally energetic, joyful, and loves the fun. But when they are not happy, they will clearly and loudly say it. These toddlers are also quite obstinate and hard to fit in regular routines.

To help them succeed:

> Acknowledge their unique temperament and understand their triggers.

> Teach them self-help skills to get going if their energy is low or how to calm down when their activity level is very high. Some simple and effective ways to calm down are counting from 1 to 10, taking deep breaths, doing jumping jacks to get rid of excess energy, and redirecting them to other activities.

> Set a daily routine that includes play and other activities that enhance their gross motor movements. Please provide them with opportunities to play and explore safely. It is necessary to childproof your home.

> Insist on nap time. An afternoon nap will refresh their body and mind, preventing mood swings and tantrums.

> Do not let them sit in front of a television or do passive activities. Break the boredom by taking them outside and play in the outdoors.

> Become a calming influence. Understand how your temperament affects their temperament and find ways to become a role model.

- Passive or Cautious Toddlers—These children prefer activities that don't require a lot of physical effort, move slower, and want to sit down more often. They are slow-to-warm-up when meeting new people and often withdraw when faced with an unfamiliar situation. They also need ample time to complete their tasks.

To help them succeed:

- ➢ If your child is less active, set guidelines or deadlines to prompt them to finish the given tasks.

- ➢ Invite them to play actively by using interesting sounds, bright toys, or gentle persuasion.

- ➢ Always accentuate the positive. Be lavish with praise and words of encouragement when they display efforts or achieve simple milestones.

- Flexible or Easy Toddlers—These children are very adaptable, generally calm, and happy. But sometimes, they are easily distracted and need a lot of reassurance and love from you.

To help them succeed:

- ➢ Be realistic and expect mood changes when something isn't smooth sailing. Don't be too hard on the child when they display unusual outburst.

➤ Please provide them with interactive activities and join him. Sometimes, it's easy to let them play their own devices because of their good-natured personality. It is necessary to introduce other options to enhance their skills.

➤ Read the signs and find out the reasons for subtle changes in the behavior and attitude toward something. Be observant and have a particular time for him.

3.

How To Stimulate Good Behavior In Children

Stimulating a good behavior in children is one of the best ways to impose limits without applying punishments regularly. The only problem is how to do that. In most cases, our little ones tested our limits and seemed to do anything not to obey.

Here are ways to stimulate good behavior:

Be the Example

Being an example in our children is the most effective way to teach anything - both good and bad. When it comes to motivate good behavior in children, it is no different. Here are a few examples of what you can do for your child to learn.

Catch your child's attention when you split snacks with your husband or when you have to wait in the bank queue, pointing out that adults also have to share and stay too.

Realize The Good Behavior

If you are like any parent in the world, when your child is behaving well, you leave him playing alone and take advantage of the time to do anything you may need to. But when your child is misbehaving, you direct all your attention to him to resolve the situation. Your attention is what kids most want to get this attention, and sometimes children will misbehave. The best way to inspire good behavior in children is to pay attention when they behave well and take your attention away when they are misbehaving. This is completely counter-intuitive for us and can be a difficult habit to cultivate. But once you get used to it, it will become easier and more comfortable.

A great way to do this is to play with your child when he is quiet in his corner and praise him when he obeys you the first time you speak.

Understand The Stage Of Development

This tip is easy to understand. Each child has a behavior; however, you cannot require three to act as the same as a child who is ten. That is, do not try to go to a three-hour lunch with your little boy hoping he will be quiet for the whole lunch. Do not want a two-year-old child not to put everything in his mouth. Each age has a phase, and there is no use to demand different behavior from a child.

Have Appropriate Expectations

Parents have high expectations. This is not wrong when expectations are possible. For example, do not expect a tired child to behave well, or a one-month-old baby to sleep through the night.

Create Structure and Routine

A child with a structured routine tends to behave better. They already know what to look forward to and are used to it. A child with a routine feels safe and thus lives more calmly. A child without a routine has a sense of insecurity that will disrupt much in the time to educate and encourage good behavior.

Uses Disciplinary Strategies

Rather than humiliating or beating children, there are positive disciplinary strategies that teach, set boundaries, and encourage good behavior in children. Some of these are: give options, put somewhere to think, talk, give affection, and a system of rewards (reward can be a simple compliment, it does not have to be gifts or food).

Understand That the Bad Behavior Worked So Far

If throwing tantrums and disobeying worked for him to get your attention so far, changing this behavior will take time. He will have to realize and understand that you will no longer pay attention to him when he behaves badly, but when he behaves well.

Instilling good behavior practices in young children is a must for any responsible parent, but sometimes it can also be quite complicated and laborious. However, beginning to instill this type of behavior as early as possible will help build a good foundation for the child's behavior and attitudes in the future.

Here are some more ideas to help parents with the task of encouraging good behavior in their children.

Models To Follow

Children tend to mirror the behaviors of parents and those with whom they coexist more closely. Therefore, be careful about your actions and language used when the child is around to avoid misunderstanding ideas and misconceptions about how you should behave towards others. This includes talking properly and conducting politely to both your partner and family and the child. Try to avoid loud, unstructured arguments when the child is around. We do not mean you can't disagree with your spouse, because the child must also be aware that these exist. But try to have the arguments always controlled and civil around children.

Be Firm

Parents should be affectionate, but still adamant about instilling discipline in their children. The child must know how to respect his parents, even when they do not have what they want. Understanding when to say "no" at the right times is an essential step in your education.

Establishing Limits

It is fundamental to establish limits, rules, and consequences for unwanted behavior. Increase limits on children to be able to distinguish right from wrong.

You started tracking your child's progress long before he left the warmth of your belly: in the tenth week, the heart began beating; on the 24th week, his hearing developed and listened to your voice; in the 30th week, he began to prepare for childbirth. Now that he or she is in your arms, you're still eager to keep up with all the signs of your little one's development and worries that he might be left behind. Nonsense! Excessive worry will not help at all, so take your foot off the accelerator and enjoy each phase. Your child will realize all the fundamental achievements of maturity. He will learn to walk, talk, potty, and when you least expect it, you will be riding a bicycle alone (and no training wheels!). He will do all only in his time.

Consider what is expected for each age just for reference. The best thing to do is to set aside the checklist of the abilities your child needs to develop and play together a lot. There is no better way to connect with and build your child than through playtime.

To help you even further realize the goals mentioned above or processes, I would like to say some tips here that stimulate a child's intellectual, motor, social, and emotional development:

Books

The parents' role is fundamental for children to learn to love reading and make books a pleasure, rather than an obligation. For 17%, the father was the one who played the role. From the third month of your child's life, you can use plastic books in the bath. From the sixth, when the baby can already carry objects to the mouth with his hands, leave cloth books in the cradle - in addition to being able to bite them, he will not be able to rip the pages! At all ages, talk about the cover, the pictures, the colors, and let the child turn the pages.

Memory

Memory is a form of storing knowledge and must be permeated by a context. Start by helping your child memorize words by showing a represented object. If you're walking on the street and crossing a bicycle, point and say, "Look, son, a bicycle." This is how he will build associations. From the first year, he will say a few words and try to repeat the names of what you show. But it is from the age of 2 that the ability to retain information increases.

Creating

Create characters and a dream of fantastic worlds. All of this is important in developing the creativity of little ones; it also contributes to problem-solving. To make the narrative more exciting, how about testing the improvisational ability of the two of you? Separate figures from objects, landscapes, colors, foods, and animals can be drawn or cut from magazines. By age 7, as the child is already literate, you can help him record your small booklets' adventures.

Always Ask

When you pick up your child from school, you always say, "How was your day?" And he says, "Cool." It was not exactly what you wanted to hear, right? To avoid generic responses, develop the questions so that the child needs to express what he thinks and justify his response. Ask: "What did you enjoy most today?" And he will be forced to grow more elaborate reasoning, requiring him to work linguistic and logical skills. At three years old, he can already relate experiences he went through and say whether those were good or bad. At 4, you can ask for details, descriptions, and colleagues who were with him.

Clap, Clap, Tum, Tum

One of the best ways to develop motor coordination is to teach rhythm to your child. To do this, use your hands. From the seventh month, clap with him to the sounds of your favorite songs, interspersing slow songs with other accelerated songs to see the difference. You will see that your baby will be able to hit his little hands.

Everything Fits

From the age of 7 months, the baby begins to hold objects; in about a year and a half, he will start to put the pieces together. Besides being a good exercise for coordination, the child will learn which part will fit within the other. For your child to love and learn from this, he can play with pots and plastic mugs while you prepare lunch. They also offer small puzzles from the age of two and a half (about six pieces).

Step By Step

Climbing stairs is a great exercise to develop agility and coarse motor coordination and help strengthen muscles. At one year of age, the child can already perform the activity, but only by placing both feet on the same step, one at a time. He will gain strength and balance with growth until, by age 3, he will probably rise by placing one foot on each step alternately. Even at this stage, he must be accompanied by an adult to avoid accidents.

Bonding & Trust

Establishing relationships of trust is essential for the development of the child. The first people he does it with are the parents. For this, one factor is necessary: never lie. If he asks if the injection will hurt, be honest, and say it will, yes, but it will pass. Tell him he's going to get wet; it's going to hurt, he's going to be cold, so he knows what to expect and learns to trust what you say.

Congratulate your child when he is good at something, encouraging him to continue. If scolding is necessary, pay close attention to how to do it. Saying "what you did was naughty" is quite different from saying, "you are naughty!" Do not let the child think that the criticized trait is part of his personality, so he will not incorporate it into his self-image.

4.

What is Discipline?

Disciplining toddlers pose significant challenges for parents. Toddlers are notorious for continually testing the boundaries set by their moms or dads. The fact that toddlers cannot communicate their feelings or thoughts becomes a real challenge for parents who want their kids to behave well or obey their instructions to prevent them from harm.

It is the parents' job to teach your child the difference between acceptable and unacceptable behaviour. Getting your child to behave the way you would like them to act is not as hard as you think. Learning takes time, and several weeks will go by when working on good behaviour before you see a change. It will be challenging, but try not to get frustrated if you don't see results right away.

What is Discipline?

Discipline is technically a method or a set of strategies used to prevent, resolve, or correct behavioural problems. The term originated from the Latin word "discipline," which means training and instruction. Its root word is "d'isere" or "to learn."

Primary Objectives of Discipline

1. Instill sound morals

2. Develop desirable behaviours

3. Modify unacceptable behaviours

4. Protect the child's emotional and mental health

5. Keep and enhance a close relationship with him

Parents use it to teach their kids about rules, guidelines, principles, expectations, and consequences. Toddlers do not have the essential skills to handle social situations or act appropriately. Parents need to guide and help their children learn desirable behaviour that will make them feel good and accepted. Discipline is not a one-time practice, but a continuing effort to develop and entrench good social habits to children.

Discipline Versus Punishment

Distinguishing the difference between discipline and punishment is critical for parents and caregivers. It is vital to remember that discipline is about teaching the child of appropriate and acceptable manners or behaviours. Punishment is about enforcing disciplinary consequences that may include spanking, verbal admonishment, and other punitive acts that hurt the child physically or emotionally.

The methods of disciplining the child vary due to cultural differences, beliefs, educational attainment of parents, customs, and values. In Western countries, the debate over corporal punishment continues, while embracing other nations turn to "positive parenting" techniques.

Over time, history displays variation in discipline methods:

- **Medieval Times**. Children during these periods were subject to corporal punishment at home and throughout society. The primary reason why parents resort to harsh discipline was to ensure that their kids would have a place in heaven.

- **Colonial Times**. The Puritans in the United States during these times practised harsh punishments, which include beating children, even for minor infractions. Young children were allowed to play freely, but older children expected to be accountable and learn adult chores.

- **Pre-Civil and Post-Civil War Times**. During this slavery era in the United States, the prevalence of corporal punishment became common among African American families. The traditional styles of parenting were affected by the violent suppression of West African cultural practices. Parents are forced to teach children to display desirable behaviour when facing white people and expect dehumanizing actions that include sexual, emotional, and physical violence. Even after the Proclamation of

34

Emancipation, which ended slavery, many Afro-American parents still used corporal punishment out of fear that if they did not, this would put their family at risk of discrimination and violence.

- **The Twentieth Century**. In the early part of the 20th century, the child-rearing experts advocated adopting proper habits in disciplining kids and abandoning the romantic view of childhood. The Infant Care, a 1914 U.S. Children's Bureau pamphlet, admonished parents who played with their babies and urged them to follow a strict schedule.

Unfortunately, up to this day, some people consider punishment and discipline synonymous. According to the Thesaurus, control is geared on self-control and regulation, while punishment is more about abuse or sentence.

But in reality, discipline is positive guidance that trains and teaches the child to develop abilities to manage his emotions and learn to make smart decisions that are acceptable to society. Whereas, punishment is about regulating or controlling the child's behaviour by injecting fear and imposing physical or emotional consequences that include spanking, hitting, name-calling, prohibiting privileges, shaming, and withholding affection. Discipline encourages the thinking brain to learn and adopt a new practice. Punishment inflicts pain or suffering for the action hoping to modify future behaviour.

Discipline teaches a child to behave according to the rules and focus on future behaviour. Punishment invokes fear of consequence to the emotional mind.

While punishment makes the child behave when you are present, it may result in the formation of behaviour that is manipulative, challenging, or defiant. Also, it can discourage him from attempting to try new things because of fear to bring disappointment, pain, or shame to the family.

To be effective, discipline must be:

- Administered by an adult who has an affective bond with the child (parents, teacher, or caregiver)

- Perceived by the child as reasonable and fair

- Consistent and appropriate for the behaviour that requires a change

- Self-enhancing or leading to becoming self-disciplined

- Temperamentally and developmentally appropriate

The primary goal of discipline is to guide the child to fit into the real world effectively and happily. It serves as the foundation of the development of self-discipline. It is not about forcing him to obey the rules, instead of teaching him what is right and what is not. Parents should make sure that while they are enforcing discipline, children should know that they love, trust, and support them. Trust is vital for adequate control. A harsh punishment that uses verbal abuse, name-calling, humiliation, or shouting will make it difficult for children to trust and respect the parents.

There is no shortcut for disciplining the child. Raising your children to become emotionally mature requires time and a significant amount of energy to teach acceptable behaviours and limits. It is a pleasure to see your child shows assertiveness without being aggressive, knows how to postpone self-gratification, tolerates discomfort when it is necessary and considerate of others' feelings or needs. All these are the outcomes of the firm and loving discipline.

An effective discipline sustains mutual respect between the parent and the child. The interventions should enforce consistently and reasonably that ensure his protection from danger and help him develop a sense of control, responsibility, self-discipline, and a healthy conscience. Any inconsistency will confuse the child, regardless of his developmental stage. It will also lessen your effectiveness as a role model or enforcer of discipline.

Some factors that affect the consistency of discipline are cultural differences between parents and disagreements on child-rearing strategies. Often, to resolve the disputes, parents seek the help of the pediatricians who can suggest practical ways to discipline the child using the principles that are supported by academic literature and research.

Discipline for Early Toddlers (1-2 years old)

At 12-18 months old, the toddler is not yet capable of controlling his response because of the undeveloped frontal lobe of the brains. This part is responsible for some aspects of emotions, along with other functions. During this stage, toddlers experience extreme emotions, crying, or acting out when tired, scared, hungry, want something, sick, overwhelmed, and need a diaper change.

Toddlers usually are experimenting and exercising their wills to gain control. It is necessary to exercise parental tolerance and enforce disciplinary interventions only when necessary to prevent destructive behaviour, limit aggression, or keep them safe.

A firm "No," a brief explanation of why it is not allowed, like "No, hot!" or removing your child from the situation, typically works. It is also important to supervise the activities of the child to make sure that the behaviour will not recur and, at the same time, show that you are not withdrawing your love and support. Young toddlers are susceptible to fear of abandonment. Often, you are at a loss of what he wants, so you need to skilful and observant to figure out what he wants.

Discipline for Late Toddlers (2-3 years old)

Your two-year-old child begins to understand and use language to express his emotions and wants. However, do not expect him to think logically, follow complicated directions, or predict his actions. He can follow simple instructions, but somehow forgets what he is doing.

During this stage, he also learns to give orders, demands, and show aggression. It is usual for toddlers to be short-tempered because of low frustration threshold and little impulse control.

A 3-year-old toddler can communicate his wishes and needs clearly, but his logical thinking skill remains underdeveloped. He often gives in and follows his impulses, but can remember simple rules. It is the period where he enjoys hearing the same stories and songs over and over again, loves routines, and learns by repeating sounds.

During this period, the struggle to be independent, assertive, and master some skills continues. When the child meets some limits, he becomes frustrated that usually leads to temper outbursts or tantrums. Parents should realize that the acts do not necessarily mean willful defiance, disobedience, or anger and understand the real reason for the behaviour.

It is necessary to continue setting routines and limits and have a realistic expectation of what they can do. Do not expect your toddler to regulate or control his behaviour by giving directions or verbal prohibitions alone. It is vital to supervise and redirect him into another activity to prevent temper flare-ups. By knowing the pattern of the child's reactions, you can avoid tantrums and other misbehaviour.

Parents need to be consistent during this time when instilling discipline. If you say NO, mean it and avoid changing your response when the child starts to throw a tantrum or whine.

The objective of disciplining your child is not to punish, but to improve the child and help them act like they are supposed to. Since child discipline, at times, is indeed one of the least fanciful aspects of parenting, the challenge that comes with it might make you want to think that it is impossible to discipline your child without punishing them. The truth is, resorting to punishment is not an excellent way to teach a lesson to your kids. You might interview some parents, and you want to confirm what pattern of discipline they use. You might hear them say: "I use them interchangeably." But the right question is, are those words synonyms? Obviously no!

But why is it that the objectives of disciplining are never to punish? When a parent punishes a child, the child would undoubtedly be physically affected. Moreover, in most cases, the brain is involved. All parents would desire a healthy mind for their kids.

Additionally, punishment is fear-based. And constant fear is not healthy for the brain. But sadly, many parents hope that threatening as part of a sentence will instill fear, and that., in turn, will discard that undesired behaviour and pick up a desired one.

Little wonder that they didn't realize that they are unknowingly messing up their kid's brain. It is capable of mental disorder, stress hormone elevation, emotion dysregulation, and externalizing behaviour. In some cases, they become bullies or victims. In sharp contrast to punishment, discipline improves a child's well-being. It allows a child to focus on the right lesson; they avoid being vindictive, distrustful, and spiteful.

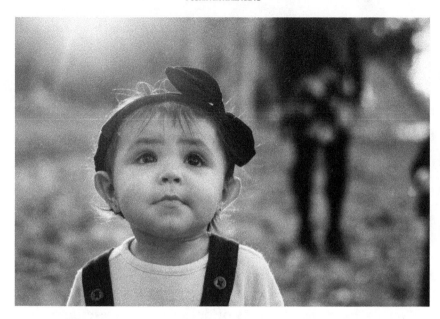

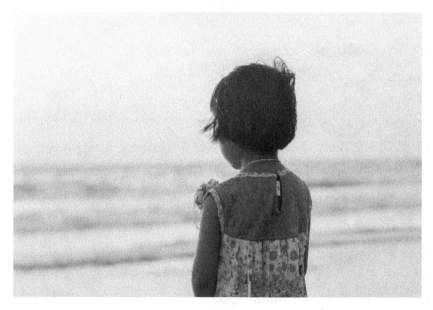

5.

Types of Discipline

Children are fantastic. They have a natural curiosity, innocence, and energy which allows them to see the world in unique ways. Toddlers are at the very beginning of a beautiful journey; to them, the world is full of new and exciting experiences. Unfortunately, toddlers and even young children aren't aware of the dangers which exist in the world around them, so it's your responsibility as a parent to guide them and keep them safe.

Discipline means creating a set of rules and guidelines to help your child grow into a healthy and considerate adult. More importantly, the domain will ensure that your child does not run into the road, randomly hit strangers, or even throw food around in a restaurant. Good discipline will allow you to go out to various places with your toddler and enjoy the experience.

Unfortunately, it is simply not possible to draw up a standard set of rules which will miraculously provide you with the perfectly behaved child. Every toddler is different. The influences and pressures placed on them will vary according to the pressure on you and your approach to each issue. The guidelines you must create and enforce will continuously be changing!

Good discipline is established by reacting positively to any situation and explaining why a specific type of behaviour is necessary. It is also beneficial for your toddler to understand that there are consequences for not behaving correctly. Likewise, results must be relative to the issue, and you must carry through with it when your toddler has continued to misbehave. If you can't enforce the consequence, your child won't have any incentive to behave respectfully. Even when it's difficult to see your child upset, you must be aware that you're thinking of their future, which is more significant than anything else.

Types of Discipline

It should now be evident that there are several different approaches to disciplining your child. There isn't one specific type which has been proven "better," and many parents will find that they have a preferred method but use a little of each approach:

Positive Parenting

It is one of the better-known approaches and is being proven to have positive effects. Oregon State University started a research project in 1984 with 206 boys, which they felt were at risk of juvenile delinquency; the children met with the researchers every year until their 33rd birthday. The research has shown that positive parenting can improve behaviour and interactions between generations.

As its name suggests, this approach to parenting and discipline relies on being favourable to your child as much as you can. As a parent, you'll seek to remain calm, regardless of the situation. In return, traditional punishments, such as removing love or toys, stay as the idea is that your child will respond to you because of the bond you have with them and because they want to.

Reward and Punishment

This approach to discipline involves creating the rules you expect your child to abide by the following. If they don't behave according to these rules, you remove an item from them for a set amount of time; this will usually be their favourite toy.

If you adopt this approach, you'll need to be consistent—once you have said you'll remove the item, you must do so. However, this can often lead to another issue. A toddler may begin to realize that this is a result of their behaviour, yet this won't stop them from being upset, and you'll then need to decide whether to comfort them or not.

Research suggests that this is the fundamental flaw with this type of parenting because most parents will not wish to remove a toy as it feels wrong. Unfortunately, if you say you're going to do something and then don't, you will have just taught your toddler that they can push it further the next time. Equally, if you remove the item and then comfort your upset child, you will be effectively rewarding their bad behaviour with comfort, which can encourage them to repeat the bad behaviour.

Reward and punishment are often referred to as "tough love." It is because it can be tough on the parent and your child.

Behaviour Modification

There is a technique that involves ignoring naughty or disrespectful behaviour. In contrast, praise and rewards are offered when your child does something right. If ignoring complaints or behaviour does not stop the action, the punishment would need to be awarded.

This approach focuses on consequences but will often overlap with the reward and punishment approach.

Emotional Discipline

Children are subject to the same range of emotional responses as adults. In many situations, they will be unsure of their feelings and how they should influence their approach. This type of discipline encourages your child to open up about their feelings. The belief is that understanding their emotions will allow them to learn how to deal with them and react positively in any situation.

Research suggests that there is merit in this approach. Children capable of dealing with emotions will generally be calmer like adults and adapt to various situations.

Commanding

It is an old-fashioned approach to parenting and is based on the premise that children should be seen and heard. Adopting this approach means that you expect your children to do as they are told. If not, then you'll immediately dish out punishment with no specific reward for good behaviour. Punishment can range from loss of toys to physical spanking.

This approach works more along the lines of fear than love. It isn't seen as an appropriate or effective long-term method, and many children who have been brought up this way will reach their teenage years and rebel against the strict rules. The result is a child who does all the things that you have taught them not to. Besides, in many cases, the relationship between parent and child is, at best strained; more likely, it's simply non-existent.

Merits of Positive Parenting

Discipline is how you guide your toddler into becoming a well-rounded child and, subsequently, a positive adult. It's generally accepted that this is the best method for teaching your toddler into adulthood whilst retaining a strong bond between you and them.

There are several merits associated with this approach:

Recognizing feelings

Your toddler is surprisingly aware of what is happening around them. If they see from a young age that you are sad when they don't follow your guidelines, they will resist doing these things. It is because they will want to keep you happy, which is a natural desire in children.

By starting this at toddler age, you will enable your child to understand how their actions affect others and consider this before they act.

Emotions

Just as your toddler will learn your feelings and how to consider others before they act, they will also react to a positive parenting approach by feeling good about themselves. It is inevitable. A toddler will see that you're happy when they respond in a certain way, which will generate additional positive attention for them. They will quickly realize that they like the feeling. In turn, you can encourage them to feel good when they achieve something.

In contrast, if you adopt a punishment-based system, you will generally find that your child doesn't decide or speak up because they don't want to incur the consequences of a wrong decision. It will stunt their emotional growth.

Personality Development

It's highly likely that you enjoy being praised. After all, everyone likes to be recognized, and so what to do as praise inspires you to try again and achieve even greater things. The same is true when you apply a positive parenting approach to your toddler. Although young, they will quickly recognize the benefits and satisfaction of reaching for something and achieving it.

Although your child is just a toddler, this can be one of the best times to start this approach. After all, they will have just started walking and are ready to try a host of new things!

Integration

Whilst you don't need to raise a child that follows the herd, you do want your child to be aware of how their actions affect others. It will allow them to develop the best approach to any issue whilst keeping most people happy. Only by adopting this approach in the adult world will they be able to achieve great success.

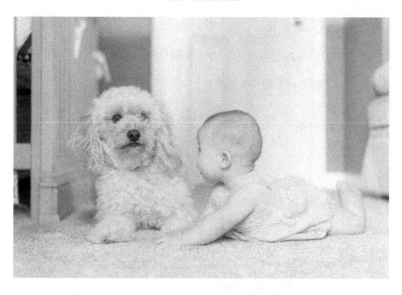

6.

Why Every Parent Should Choose to Parent Positively

P ositive parenting has been around for hundreds of years. It is seen in the action's parents take to help their kids set positive goals. It is seen in the support we give our children and even as we try to relate to them. These are all tremendous positive principles of parenting. The essential changes between then and now is that children were often told what to do and how to do it by their parents, but never really given a reason why. They just knew to do what they were told, or they may be punished or spanked. That is the beauty of positive parenting; it teaches kids the "why" behind the actions they are told to perform. Parents back then controlled their kids more than they dedicated themselves to training them to see fit.

It's Never Too Late to Start Positive Parenting

Positive parenting not only impacts your child's life in affirmative ways, but it changes the life of the parent as well. When conducted properly, this method of parenting builds a solid foundation to heighten self-esteem and positively driven emotions between both the parent(s) and the child. It has been proven by various health professionals, family counsellors, and psychiatrists that the relationship between the parents raising kids grows positively as well when implementing these practices. There is less stress when one parent does not have to worry about using heavy-hand or harmful techniques. Trust is heightened, and issues that arise are seen more as opportunities than negative obstacles.

Children Are People Too

There are many simple tricks that, if we were merely able to change our mindset, will work wonders when it comes to discipline. Much of what you'll learn throughout the chapters in this book are simple things that will make you wonder why you hadn't thought and utilized them before now. Many benefits come along with being a positive parent. I will tell you that there, not an easy way out that it takes hard work and dedication to practice and utilize this style of parenting properly. But I assure you, there is a range of both short and long-term benefits that you and your children will positively grow from these!

Benefits of Positive Parenting

Positive parenting, by no means, lacks discipline. While as a parent, you still need to correct wrong behaviour, there are different things you can do to do this without yelling, hitting, etc. successfully. It is where learning about positive parenting can quickly become one of the best parenting decisions you'll ever make!

Secure Attachment

They should secure attachment is the foundation for healthy development in all children. It allows the healthy building of resilience for how your child is to act during their time as an adult. It also helps in superb brain development. To understand this, we must get scientific for a brief moment. The human brain doesn't mature until we are in our twenties. Our first 3-6 years of life on this planet are crucial for the further development of our centre of command.

Ability to Understand Feelings

Positive parenting thrives on the fact that you can share feelings between you and your kids openly. For example, if your child decides to run across a parking lot without looking at their surroundings first, and calmly explain to them how that action makes you nervous and how upset you would be if they were injured in any way. They will follow your directions because they don't want you to be sad if they get hurt. This type of behaviour from a parenting standpoint builds empathy between you and your child that will last a lifetime. It will also teach your child to think about the feelings of others before acting.

Decrease of Power Struggles

Disciplining your kids in harsh manners can cause them to feel shameful and poorly about themselves. They bury all that shame of their lousy behaviour within themselves instead of merely correcting it, which fuels them to act out in ways parents don't see fit continuously. If you continue down this path with your child, they will see you as an obstacle, which will result in power struggles. It's crucial to set up boundaries but do so with empathy and fairness in mind. If you maliciously treat your kids, they will grow up thinking it's okay to treat others that way too.

Healthy Emotional Development

When children grow up feeling good about themselves, they will mature into someone that has good self-esteem. They know they are easily capable of success with hard work and can truly feel good about positive accomplishments. Using harsh punishments can plant a sense of fear and shame that will later grow into them, making bad decisions or surpassing, making crucial decisions at all.

Uncover Motivations

It is known that all of us are motivated by different things. Children are human too, so this applies to them as well. As a parent, you only limit yourself when you use harsh punishments. If anything, you think more creatively through the means of positive parenting. When you learn how to isolate the things your child values, you can then use that to your advantage.

Building Strong Relationships

Positive parenting can allow plenty of room for positive relationships between family members to flourish since they are based on accomplishments and good memories. Parents must learn how boundaries are to be set through loving guidance. It builds a circle of respect for everyone in the family. When done correctly, parents will no longer have to discipline children but offer advice when they need it.

Development of Character

It is through the means of lively parenting sprouts children who are motivated by the desire for excellence in their lives. They wish to behave well to truly reach their goals, not because they fear being punished if they don't do as such. It says that when they grow up, they can watch their results and themselves as it seeks opportunities to do well in all the things they do.

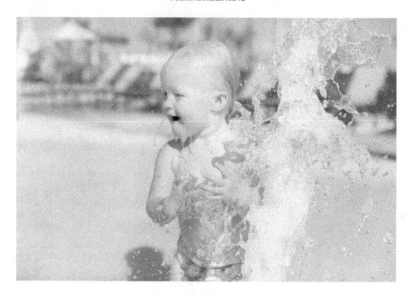

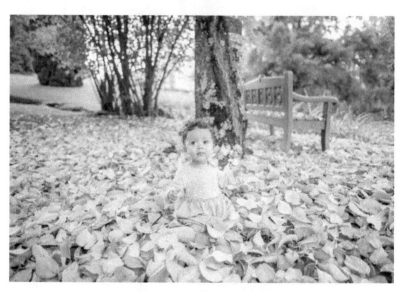

7.

The Positive Discipline to Instill in Your Child

It is vital to reinforce the objectives of Positive Discipline, remembering that it is about teaching essential life and social skills in manners that are encouraging and respectful to both the learners (children) and mentors (parents, teachers, caregivers, childcare providers). It is based on the concept that discipline must be taught to children with kindness and firmness, neither permissive nor punitive.

To make Positive Discipline more effective, it is necessary for parents, teachers, and other adult influences to create a nurturing environment that meets all the basic needs of the child, such as food, shelter, and clothing, extending to non-physical needs such as love, encouragement, and acceptance.

- Parental love is about the unconditional love that is acted out by providing care and gentle guidance, giving time and attention to children, and resolving any social conflict.

- Acceptance makes children feel that no matter what they do, whether wrong or right, they are loved.

56

- Encouragement is showing support in concrete ways that help children figure out how to avoid or correct mistakes, including finding their strengths to pursue passions and life goals.

In a nutshell, parents are the primary support of children who ensure their positive growth and development.

Positive Discipline at Home

Discipline begins at home. As early as possible, kids are taught to be responsible for their actions and distinguish right from wrong. Positive Discipline at home uses healthy and positive interactions to prevent inappropriate acts or behavioural problems before they begin and become habits. It teaches kids the correct behaviour and be respectful through appreciation, encouragement, consequences, and other non-violent strategies.

The outcomes are:

- Children do better when there is routine, consistency, and lots of positive encouragement.

- A positive relationship with parents dramatically reduces the occurrence of challenging behaviour.

- A non-punitive discipline that provides significant long-term benefits compared to punishment.

- Children respond positively to parents or caregivers whom they trust. It is essential to use the strategies consistently by all caregivers.

Creating a Safe Environment

Childproof your home and supervise his movements to see that he is safe while exploring his immediate surroundings.

Establishing a Routine

Routines help children perform or behave appropriately because they know the expectations of their parents. A specific way to guarantee optimum care, safety, and enjoyment will help your child feel secure, more in control, and less anxious, hence developing strong self-discipline.

Planning Ahead

If you have to run errands and need to take your child with you, it is necessary to talk to him and let him know your expectations of his behaviours. It will prepare him and try his best to behave well. However, for little children who do not fully comprehend yet what you are trying to say, better have toys, crayons, books, and other activity tools with you when you go out to keep him occupied while shopping, waiting for the doctor's appointment, or travelling.

Having Clear Expectations

Discuss your expectation with your child. If you set 5 expectations like-Be Kind, Be Respectful, Be Responsible, Be Helpful, and Be Safe, do not forget to tell them. Have a conversation with him about the acts and deeds that demonstrate your expectations. Make sure that you also display those acceptable behaviours because your child is always watching your examples.

Offering Choices

Choices that are suitable for his age will help him gain a sense of independence and self-control. By offering options, you empower him to become more decisive and stand up for what he believes is right for him. It also applies to the consequences of misbehaviour or disobeying your rules. Make him choose between two safe, logical values that aim to give him a lesson and a warning not to repeat the mistake. Always follow through and enforce the consequence to make him see that you are serious about Discipline.

Building a Positive Relationship

Spending quality time with your child reinforces your relationship, helping him develop a strong sense of belonging, significance, and connection. Allow him to choose the activity or topic. It also lessens the occurrence of misbehaviour because he does not want to disappoint you.

Redirecting the Negative Behaviour

Maybe your child is bored, or for whatever reason, he starts acting out. It is essential to provide a suitable alternative that will stop him from misbehaving and enjoy himself. Always see to it that your child is well-rested, well-fed, and engaged in stimulating and fun activity. Redirecting his sudden malicious behaviour to another activity that interests him will generate appropriate action.

Calm Down Before You Address Misbehaviour

Do not try to discipline your child when you are angry, frustrated, or experiencing physical or mental fatigue because you will lose your objectivity. Calm yourself first and take a time out to steady your nerves. It will help you think clearly and handle the situation somewhat yet firmly.

Being Firm and Kind at the Same Time

It is the positive Discipline in its best form. You respond to each situation or misbehaviour with kindness and respect to your child, but firm enough to impose the consequences. It is also essential to let your child explain and justify his acts, but no matter how convincing his reason, make him understand that rules are rules. Remind him that you set limits for a purpose- to keep him safe and prevent mistakes that may hurt him or others. If he chooses to defy any of them, he needs to face the consequences of his actions.

Catch Him Being Good

Do not let good deeds go unnoticed. Whenever you observe your child behaving properly, appreciate his efforts, so he is aware that he is doing well.

Distinguishing Factors Between Normal Behaviour and Misbehaviour

What keep you thinking that your child is displaying misbehaviour or expected behaviour? It is necessary to have truthful expectations about your kid's behaviour, considering the stage of his development. Every step has distinct challenges that trigger actions, which you can mistakenly view as intentional misbehaviour. By understanding these stages, you will know the difference.

Here are some examples of typical or developmentally appropriate behaviour:

Example No. 1:

• Developmentally Appropriate or Normal Behaviour: Tantrums

• Developmental Tasks: The child is beginning to handle his frustrations and throws tantrums when upset and does not understand why he needs to do something. A classic example is when he does not want to brush his teeth or go to bed early.

61

Example No. 2:

• Developmentally Appropriate or Normal Behaviour: Energetic and Active

• Developmental Tasks: The need to explore and discover. One manifestation is the difficulty of sitting quietly for a long time, like during church attendance or storytelling period.

Example No. 3:

• Developmentally Appropriate or Normal Behaviour: Independent

• Developmental Tasks: He wants to do things on his own like feeding himself, choosing clothes to wear, or picking the toys he wants to play.

Example No. 4:

• Developmentally Appropriate or Normal Behaviour: Being talkative

• Developmental Tasks: He becomes curious about everything around him, so he asks many questions. His vocabulary is also growing, so he is excited to use the words he learns.

When your child is misbehaving:

• Hault whatever you are doing and give your full attention to your child.

• Remain calm and speak with your normal voice tone.

• If out in a public area, remove him from the situation that triggers his emotional outburst.

• Get down to his eye level.

• Make him understand what you feel before reminding your child about your expectations from him. "I know that you still want to play, but it is time to go home."

• Discuss the expected behaviour and asks him what he needs to do about it.

• State the consequence for the misbehaviour.

• Follow through with the result.

• Acknowledge when you see your child correcting his behaviour.

• Reconnect and restore your relationship through affection, hugs, or plays.

Dealing with a little child can be tiring and challenging, so do not forget to take care of yourself. It is a must to find time for yourself and find support when necessary.

- Eat a healthy diet and exercise regularly.

- Spend time in nature or have a "me" time to relax.

- Engage in activities that make you feel good and happy. Do them regularly.

- Keep in touch with family and friends.

- Say no to extra responsibilities.

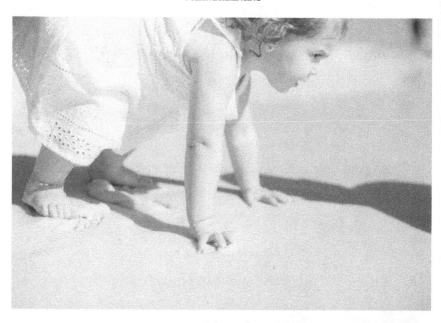

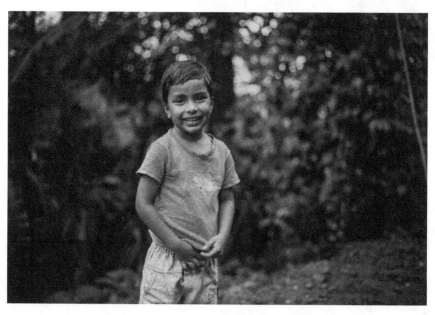

8.

Disciplining Children—How to Be a Better Parent

One of the best difficulties of child-rearing is teaching children. Between the periods of toddlerhood (around two) and approximately ten, children are wipes. They learn and assimilate everything around them. They copy their good examples and endeavour to emulate conduct, they have their quarrels and spats and emergencies, and they're just steadily going to the conviction that the world does not rotate around them.

Furthermore, your activity as a parent is to support them, direct them, value them, and discipline children when they need it. It's never simple disciplining children, yet you ought to recollect that the motivation behind disciplining children is to teach, and uphold limits, to adjust conduct. It's not to rebuff, it's not to menace, and it's not to lash out in dissatisfaction (however, every parent will get disappointed with their children sooner or later). You will probably give the social limits and anticipated conduct into your tyke, regardless of the amount they appear to the article.

It Starts With Rules

Your children request steadiness throughout everyday life. If you've at any point asked why they'll happily watch a similar video for a long time after day, that is a piece of it. Making things unsurprising to their brief timeframe skylines is what they're doing, and they anticipate that you should be unsurprising.

Consistency originates from defining rules and limits. Grown-ups realize that they can't do all that they need; children are as yet learning this exercise (frequently over and over, and with no natural elegance to it, to be gruff). It's your activity in disciplining children to ensure that rules are established, that limits are set, and that disrupting the norms is expensive. Children are as yet finding out about activities and outcomes; if you've at any point snapped your teeth at children's TV, that lectures toward the end with the nuance of a jackhammer, which is the explanation behind it. Your children must be given house rules, they should have those rules disclosed to them, the outcomes must be appeared for breaking them, and they should have the connection between disrupting the norm and the discipline clarified.

To make house rules, pursue these tips:

1. It would help if you had a rundown that is short enough that your children will recall them. Three to four rules are useful for babies to first graders; around ten is sensible for a long time seven and up. The states ought to be SIMPLE, similar to "No hitting" and "No running in the house."

2. Those rules should be disclosed to everybody on the double. Ask for inquiries, and answer them. Clarify what the rules mean, and afterwards, have your children tell them back to you as a perception check.

3. These rules should be posted in an area where everybody can see them, even little children. Yet, they should know where the rules' writ is.

Rewards as Well As Rules

Disciplining children is more than making rules to pursue; they need affirmation and reinforcement when they comply with the laws. With no positive reinforcement, rules without anyone else will rapidly be viewed as subjective and uncalled. You'll have an emergency staring you in the face. Children work amazingly well about compensating them for practices. Make those prizes express and gain the ground towards the reward visual and self-evident. Take a stab at setting up an outline with the names of your children on the left-hand side, and the rules that you need them to comply with over the top; each time your kid complies with a standard (like "heads to sleep without a complain"), put a star on the graph, and reveal to them for what reason they're getting it. Express gratitude toward them, since that will give a prompt reinforcement. At the point when the whole outline gets filled, they get something uncommon.

What can be 'something exceptional'? It can be about anything understandable, yet they needn't be detailed.

About anything can do—here's a rundown of demonstrated prizes.

- I am getting to pick what the family has for sweet for that night.

- ome PC amusement or TV time.

- A play day with Mommy and Daddy.

- You are going out—to a child's family café, a motion picture, or the recreation centre.

- Pulling a money box toy out (you stock up a container with some toys from the Dollar Store early for this)

- Another book or being perused an old most loved one.

- A visit from their companions, or a sleepover.

- I am getting to pick what amusement the family plays on family diversion night.

It is only a glimpse of something more substantial regarding remunerating exemplary conduct. The reward is as significant as the rules in disciplining children.

At the point when your kid disrupts the guidelines (they will—it's a piece of testing limits for them, and is a piece of an effective learning process), it's your activity disciplining children as a parent to disclose to them what rule they broke, have them recognize that they defied the norm, and distribute discipline. You ultimately should be quick and firm on this; disciplining children ought to be ready, with the goal that it strengthens activities and outcomes. It may not, as your children dissent, be reasonable. However, it should be quick and have a constrained court of claims. (One thing children will attempt to get the two guardians to give different rules is gaming the framework).

When you're disciplining children, and clarify what rule was broken, sit at their dimension. Look. Have them recognize the standard and that they broke it. At that point, convey discipline.

Traditional disciplines for disciplining children can fluctuate from having a toy removed for a period to breaks. When the regulation is made, you have to rehash the standard that was broken, have them recognize the rule. Afterward, you have to embrace them and reveal to them that regardless of you cherish them. At that point, let them recount to their side of the story. The point here is that you, as the parent, are the person who sets the rules and dispenses equity; however, that no infraction of a standard will at any point cost them your affection, which is their most profound dread.

Prevent Your Toddler from Hitting Other Children

When babies are predictable about anything, it is that they are eccentric. The odds are high that your little heavenly attendant will eventually get baffled and hit somebody yet or another. It could be one of their companions. In any case, the causes and arrangements are the equivalents. Presented below are a couple of tips prevent your little child from hitting.

Tip Number 1: Do not enable the situation to transform into a joke or a diversion. Your kid likely ended up baffled since they believed they couldn't get the point they were attempting to make. They are just barely building up their communication skills.

Regardless of whether the situation seems interesting to you, don't giggle or overlook it. Hitting can rapidly transform into a genuine issue. It would help if you told the youngster, without reservation, that hitting isn't alright and not permitted. Try not to change the situation into something the kid will need to rehash to make you snicker once more. Children love consideration regardless of how they get it.

Tip Number 2: Never, ever, ever hit them back or permit another person to raise it. A few people endeavour to give the situation a chance to resolve itself by giving the children "a chance to fight it out." It does not work to stop the conduct over the long haul. Restoring the hit is fulfilling and fortifying the terrible behaviour.

Tip Number 3: Set up different ways for your tyke to impart. Children are generally hit as methods for communication and not out of outrage. They are merely attempting to constrain the world into what they need it to be. If your kid has begun hitting, invest energy-demanding those are finding different approaches to convey and request what they genuinely require. The hit was a strategy to get consideration from the other party. Demonstrate the different tyke approaches to get that consideration without hitting. It can be as straightforward as urging them to offer the other kid a toy instead of running them. Doing this can fortify that there are better approaches to get the outcomes they need.

Tip Number 4: Always investigate the whole situation. It might be that your tyke conveys fine and dandy without hitting as long as they are all around rested or not over-animated. If you focus on setting the hitting scenes, you stand a superior possibility of keeping them from happening in any case.

Tip Number 5: Be alert for potential hitting situations. When your tyke will come in a worldwide hit when with a specific gathering, you can make a routine about watching them all the more near endeavour to find out what caused the youngster's dissatisfaction. You would then be able to prevent the hitting situation from creating in any case. You can even advance in to stop the hit in mid-procedure if you are ready enough.

Tip Number 6: Sometimes, you need to expel them from the situation. When the issue has heightened to the point where the tyke is not calling it quits and empowering better communication isn't working, you may need to expel them from the situation. It is an excellent use for the standard "break" discipline technique.

Tip Number 7: Insist that your tyke apologizes for hitting. It isn't the kind of consideration they were searching for and, for the most part, functions admirably to demoralize rehashing the action.

You are never going to have the option to keep your kid from regularly hitting anybody. It is something that children do. You can, anyway, set up a situation where the youngster learns and make an effort not to rehash the conduct.

9.

Things to Consider When Disciplining Toddlers

Many parents attest to the reality that disciplining a toddler is like facing constant uphill battles. These little bundles of delight can turn to too stubborn kids who test the patience limits of caregivers and adults around them.

It is also the phase of childhood where they begin to assert their independence. One of their first words is "No," affirming the toddlers' love to do things in their way. They enjoy running away to escape. Typical toddlers are full of energy. They run, jump, play, explore, and discover everything that interests them. They love to use the sense of touch, exploring things with their feelings. Because toddlers are easily stimulated by what they see or hear, their impulsive nature can make them clumsy and touch things. Parents need to teach their children safe ways to touch or handle things and not touch hot objects.

Although raising a toddler entails a lot of hard work, seeing your child grows and develops his skills is fascinating. However, because of the developmental changes that rapidly happen during the toddler stage, it is necessary to use a disciplinary approach to foster the child's independence while teaching him socially appropriate behaviour and other positive traits.

There is an assumption that parenting techniques apply to all too often, and the kids will react or respond in a similar pattern. But every child has his own set of traits. They are in his DNA, which he inherited from his parents. Some toddlers are shy or even-tempered, while others are outgoing and have aggressive natures.

By understanding the child's unique personality and natural behaviour, you can help him adjust to the real world. It is necessary to work with his character and not against it, considering the following factors you need to consider when disciplining your toddler. Giving proper care and nourishment, providing positive and healthy activities, and instilling positive discipline is vital to his physical, mental, emotional, social, and behavioural growth.

Temperament and Behaviour

Temperament is defined as the heritable and biologically based core that influences the style of approach and response of a person. The child's early temperament traits usually predict his adult temperament.

The child's behaviour is the outcome of his temperament and the progress of his emotional, cognitive, and physical development. It is influenced by his beliefs about himself, about you, and the world in general. While it is inborn and inherent, there are specific ways to help your toddler manage it to his advantage.

Nine dimensions or traits related to temperament:

1. The activity level pertains to the amount of physical motion that your toddler demonstrates while engaged in some activities. It also includes his inactive periods.

   - Is your child a restless spirit who cannot sit still for so long or want to move around?

   - Is your toddler the quiet, little one who enjoys playing alone or watching TV?

2. Rhythmicity means the predictability or unpredictability of physical and biological functions, including hunger, bowel movement, and sleeping.

   - Does your child thrive on routine and follow regular eating or sleeping patterns?

   - Does he display unpredictable behaviour and dislike practice?

3. Attention span and persistence are the skills to remain focused on the activity for a certain period.

   - Does your toddler stick to complete a task?

   - Is he easily frustrated and look for another activity?

4. Initial Response (Approach or Withdrawal) refers to the reaction to something new and unfamiliar. It describes his initial feelings to a stimulus like a new person, place, toy, and food. His response is shown by his mood or facial expressions like smiling or motor activity, such as reaching for a toy or swallowing food. Negative reactions include withdrawal, crying, fussing, pushing away, or spitting the food.

- Is he wary or reluctant around unfamiliar situations or strangers?

- Does he welcome new faces and adjust comfortably with new settings?

5. The intensity of the reaction is associated with the level of response to any event or situation. Toddlers respond differently to events around them. Some shrieks with happiness or giggle joyfully, others throw fits, and many barely react to what is happening.

- Do you always experience trying to guess the reaction of your child over something?

- Does your child explicitly show his emotions?

6. Adaptability is the child's ability to adjust himself to change over time.

    • Is your child capable of adjusting himself to sudden changes in plans or disruptions of his routine?

    • Does he find it difficult to cope with changes and resist it as much as he can?

7. Distractibility is the level of the child's willingness to be distracted. It relates to the effects of an outside stimulus on your child's behaviour.

    • Can your child focus on his activity despite the distraction that surrounds him?

    • Is he unable to concentrate when people or other activities are going on in the environment?

8. Quality of mood is related to how your child sees the world in his own eyes and understanding. Some react with acceptance and pleasure while other children scowl with displeasure just "because" they feel like it.

    • Does he display mood changes always?

    • Does he generally have a happy disposition?

9. Sensory Threshold is linked to sensitivity to sensory stimulation. Children sensitive to stimulation require a careful and gradual introduction to new people, experiences, or objects.

    • Is your child easily bothered by bright lights, loud sounds, or food textures?

    • Is he undisturbed with such things and welcome them as such?

Active or Feisty Toddlers

These children have a tremendous amount of energy, which they show even while inside their mothers' uterus, like lots of moving and kicking. As an infant, they move around, squirm, and crawl all over the place. As toddlers, they climb, run, jump, and even fidget a lot to release their energy. They become excited while doing things or anxious around strangers or new situations.

They are naturally energetic, joyful, and loves fun. But when they are not happy, they will clearly and loudly say it. These toddlers are also quite obstinate and hard to fit in regular routines.

To help him succeed:

    • Acknowledge his unique temperament and understand his triggers.

- Teach him self-help skills to get going if his energy is low or calm down when his activity level is very high. Some simple and effective ways to calm down are counting from 1 to 10, taking deep breaths, jumping jacks to get rid of excess energy, and redirecting him to other activities.

- Set a daily routine that includes play and other activities that enhance his gross motor movements. Provide him with opportunities to play and explore safely. It is necessary to childproof your home.

- Insist on nap time. An afternoon nap will refresh his body and mind, preventing mood swings and tantrums.

- Do not let him sit in front of a television or do passive activities. Break the boredom by taking him outside and play in the outdoors.

- Become a calming influence. Understand how your temperament affects his temperament and find ways to become a role model.

- Passive or Cautious Toddlers—These children prefer activities that do not require a lot of physical effort, move slower, and want to sit down more often. They are slow-to-warm-up when meeting new people and often withdraw when faced with an unfamiliar situation. They also need ample time to complete their tasks.

To help him succeed:

- If your child is less active, set guidelines or deadlines to prompt him to finish the given tasks.

- Invite him to play actively by using interesting noises, bright toys, or gentle persuasion.

- Always accentuate the positive. Give praise and words of encouragement when they display efforts or achieve simple milestones.

- Flexible or Easy Toddlers—These children are very adaptable, generally calm, and happy. But sometimes, they are easily distracted and need a lot of reassurance and love from you.

To help him succeed:

- Be realistic and expect mood changes when something is not smooth-sailing. Do not be too hard on the child when he displays unusual outburst.

- Provide him with interactive activities and join him. Sometimes, it is easy to let him play his own devices because of his good-natured personality. It is necessary to introduce other options to enhance his skills.

- Read the signs and find out the reasons for subtle changes in the behaviour and attitude toward something. Be observant and have a special time for him.

10.

Successful Ways to Discipline Toddlers

When you have youngsters, it is advantageous just as unpleasant, and you should figure out how to train toddlers when you can. It will guarantee that they gain since the beginning what they may or may not be able to. Toddlers are a challenge every day as they find out about the world and the confinement points and limits they can push. Your child-rearing aptitudes will be tried; however, you will see incredible outcomes with excellent tyke discipline strategies.

It would help if you secured that you get familiar with the straightforward method of exact order; your little child is at a period of honesty. You should instruct them that their activities will have results not exclusively to themselves yet, additionally to other people. For particular order to work, you should empower your little child and never rebuff, or control. Your baby will form into a minding kid with the proper measure of order, and your home will be a cherishing tranquil one. You will require a flexible arrangement of guidelines and ability, you need to train toddlers, and if you are clear about this. It will make it simpler.

The control intends to instruct, train, and teach, which is exceptionally valid; your baby should be shown these things at an in all respects at an early age. Attention and results should be educated. Even though, you will love giving your little child's thoughtfulness. They have to realize when it can and when it isn't. Your youngster discipline techniques should be firm, however, sufficiently straightforward for your small child to get it. You should force outcomes, yet ones that your minor child will get it. Toddlers react to limits, and even though they will push them, they improve to having structure and limitations.

Rewarding your little child for ethical conduct is a fantastic method to train them; they will, before long, discover that they possibly get the reward when they are great. Realizing when to utilize a discipline can be a test for you. Focus on beneficial things your little child is doing and not the terrible things. However, this is more difficult than expected. Typical results help you with discipline toddlers; they will help them learn they have fouled up without you venturing in.

It would help if you located a happy medium between your little child understanding what they have fouled up and forcing an excessively harsh discipline. Even though you should recognize terrible conduct, you should endeavour to disregard it. Toddlers will respond better if they are compensated for their bad behaviour

Your tyke discipline strategies should be a great idea to do this. At the same time, there will be circumstances when your little child accomplishes something wrong if you discipline toddlers appropriately;

at that point, they will before long start to demonstrate advance. Before long, your baby will comprehend that their shrewd direct isn't accomplishing anything; they aren't getting consideration from you by any stretch of the imagination. Youngsters are incredibly sharp, and it doesn't take them long to comprehend the ideal approach to earn rewards from you.

11.

Three Keys to Calm and Effective Discipline

One of the hardest things about early parenting (or perhaps any parenting), especially when it comes to tantrums, is discipline. It's impossible to write a book about avoiding tantrums without addressing discipline alongside the communication topics we have already covered.

Hopefully, you will find it helpful that I have researched far and wide on this tricky concept and have a few conclusions. The following images have worked for many of the families I have coached and for us.

Here are the three keys to successful discipline when it involves your child:

1. Discipline is best used as a teaching tool, not a punishment

For that reason, discipline is most successful when the child's negative actions are logical, natural consequences. If we teach our children that they shouldn't misbehave because if they do, scary or painful punishments may happen, we automatically pit them against us in their developmental journey. We are also not mirroring real life. In real life, if we forget to pay rent, a car doesn't hit us. We get a fine and eventually kicked out of the apartment. Consequences for our children need to be logical and as close to natural as possible.

Instead of punishing our toddlers, we need to enlist them as coworkers in their development. To do this, we can use discipline to help them learn the difference between appropriate and inappropriate behaviour.

For example, let's say your toddler willfully throws a block at your dog's head after you have explained (for the thousandth time) that that is not allowed (can you tell I'm writing from experience?). If you throw him in his room alone for a 'time out,' it doesn't have a direct link to his behaviour. It teaches him that sometimes he will be locked away, or love and companionship will be withdrawn if his behaviour doesn't fit your liking. Since connection and friendship are the mainstays for children, this causes his foundation of love to be shaken.

In time, the damage that this causes to the relational attachment bonds in his heart will cause him to believe lies about who he is. Either he will make his whole life about doing the "right" thing, afraid that he will cause people to withdraw love and connection makes a wrong move, or he will conclude that regardless of what he does, the attachment will be removed from him for inexplicable and unpredictable reasons. This could cause him to become rebellious and reckless in his disregard for the rules.

So, in the block throwing, it makes more sense for the consequence to be that the block is taken away for some time. Now, the way that this happens matters.

As the parent in this situation, if I yank the block away and say, "No! Now you can't play with that anymore," there is no link being made that gives my child an idea of avoiding this situation in the future.

I'll have a better chance of teaching him how to navigate and reason his way through if I take his hands in mine, get down on his level, and make eye contact. I might say something like, "It's against the rules to throw the dog's block. The rules are here to keep everyone safe. That can hurt her (insert the sign language sign for 'hurt' here). She feels scared when you do that (insert sign for 'scared' here). Please tell her you are sorry (insert sign for 'sorry' here)." Then I might ask him to show her how he can pet her gently. That is a way for him to make amends for the action. The last thing I might do would be to say something like, "since you broke the rule and you threw the block at her, you won't get to play with the blocks again for a while." He might be upset at this point, but I might say something like, "You seem frustrated (insert sign for 'frustrated' here). It's hard to lose the toy you are playing. That's just what happens, though, if we throw the block at the dog and break the rules. So maybe next time you might choose not to throw the block at her, and you will be able to keep playing with the union."

Now, smaller babies will often do things like this by accident, in which case it isn't a cause for discipline, but guidance. If a baby cannot understand consequences (typically under the age of 14-16 months), redirection is your best friend. It's still a good thing in those cases to explain the rules and why we don't throw the block at the dog. However, it's typically not helpful to discipline unless the child is consciously doing malicious behaviour. Redirection is more appropriate if the offence is committed without understanding.

2. Discipline and guidance must be consistent – it's all about the long game!

Babies and toddlers learn by repetition. Thus, it requires a significant amount of patience and consistency on the parents or caregivers when helping tiny humans develop. In the scenario above, this behaviour is likely going to occur more than once. Most toddlers test the limits and boundaries over time set for them to decide how to behave in the long run.

If my child and I had that particular interaction from the previous example one time, and then the next time he does the same thing, and I don't respond in the same way, he will be confused. He may think that somehow he influenced or had some control over how I handled the situation. If I let him continue to hurt the dog, I reinforce the ideas that:

1. It's ok to break the dog,

2. The rules sometimes don't apply,

3. He doesn't always have consequences to his rule-breaking actions.

So, will he be likely to repeat this behaviour more often? Probably. Will he also become more aggressive in trying to break other rules? Very likely.

Now, as parents and caregivers, we all have rough days. We have those days where we can't exert energy for yet one more "talk" with the little one about rules or what is allowed. Or maybe even the consequences are a detriment to us (i.e., the toddler throws the toy that keeps them busy while we balance the checkbook, and we don't want to take it away because we need that time to focus. Am I the only one?).

So don't shame yourself if you are having one of those moments. Maybe redirect to a safer set of toys that can't hurt anyone while you get your work done. However, know that your overall track record of consistency is what regulates your child's understanding of what rules of conduct are and what is right vs. wrong. Overall, you want them to see that corresponding consequences will happen, for the most part, when those rules are violated. It's about what your child learns over time that will stick with him or her.

3. Get on the Same Team

Let's go back to the previous concept of working side-by-side with one another instead of head-to-head against each other. Keeping with the idea of discipline as a teaching tool rather than punishment, it's essential as parents should be to empower and work with our children. If, at any point, we are head to head working AGAINST them, we are not only less likely to get the desired behaviour we are looking for, but we are more likely to make our parenting much harder. It is because children who do not see an advocate in their parent will continue; they will fight back harder as they grow older and more vital.

One of the best tools I have found to maintain a working relationship with my toddler through his most challenging behavioural situations, is to offer to help him when he is having a hard time doing what I ask him to do.

For instance, let's say that I tell my toddler it is time to clean up. To help that transition, I usually give him a couple of minutes' notice and say something like, "just to let you know, we will need to clean up in about two minutes, so go ahead and pick one more thing to do." Then after two minutes is up, I would say it's time to clean up now and ask him to start putting his toys in the bin. If he starts to walk (or run!) out of the room instead, I would stop him and decide how to handle it.

Instead of punishing or disciplining him right then, knowing he is a toddler who is still learning, I might say something like, "I can see you are having a hard time listening to me and cleaning up your toys. I'll help you." At that point, he is much more likely to help. So I would take his hand, and we would clean up together.

If he is still resistant, then I would use some redirection tactic. I might engage him in putting away the yellow blocks while I put away the blue ones. If the child is younger than 3, it is appropriate for the adult to clean up as the child. I might also play a game with it – we might pretend that the toy box is the goal, and we get points for every stuffed animal we toss in. This is a crucial moment to be coworkers in doing the right behaviours. In this instance, punishment doesn't make sense because it doesn't reinforce the proper action, which is to listen to the parent and do what they are asked to do. But it does support a negative stigma and feeling that will now be attached to that particular request the parent makes. If I use a scary or painful punishment in this situation, the next time I ask my child to clean up, he is most likely to remember it has been a negative situation and not very likely to change his behaviour motivated by fear.

Whatever discipline as teaching technique you use, be consistent and believe in what you are doing. Believe in the long game! Suppose you consistently act on your disciplinary convictions. In that case, you will be more likely to remain calm since you already know how you want to respond to those teaching opportunities. This will be better all around for you and for your child's development.

12.

Tips to Help Your Toddler Grow Up Happy

I s it challenging to be a mom? Fresh parents aren't carrying a book. It's our responsibility to do the best care job we can do. And this is a huge responsibility. A child was born with a clear mind and a clear conscience. The people guide them around them. Self-esteem depends on how the parents and primary caregivers treat themselves, their siblings, and them. That is so significant! Here are some tips for helping your child grow well, happy, and secure:

- Be aware that treating your child with respect and understanding is the most critical thing you can do for him/her. They study all the time. We should give them limits (which they need), without their self-respect being taken away.

- When they have something to say, listen to them.

- Inspire them to learn something new, or to get a job finished.

- Include those decisions in family decisions that affect them. In terms of rights, they are equal to us. They are all tiny humans.

- Teach them how to tell the truth of what happens to them. Teach the kids how to connect, and everyone gets an opportunity to express themselves.

- Again, note that a child's self-esteem level affects all their emotions, feelings, acts, and consequences for the rest of their life. Be tender with your affection, and be kind.

Having a parent is one of the best roles a human may have. Having acceptable parenting practices is essential to help your child grow up into a positive and self-reliant adult. Feeling good about yourself is necessary to be a happier person and a prosperous one in life. Your child has typical struggles and critiques to go through. To help them understand their imperfections, you have to consider positive parenting strategies and appreciate the qualities that make them unique. Here are some matters you can say to encourage them to grow up.

You are Destined to Be Unique

Naturally, some people take a look at what other people lack. This causes jealousy and envy, which isn't right. Rather than focusing on comparing your kids, just be thankful for whom they are. Think of them as unique people who have their way of making themselves stand out. Cheer and appreciate their distinctive talents.

Know Your Assets

Let them see it after you've realized just how good your kids are. A good way is to sit with them, get a pen and paper, and write down their properties. Help them know what kind of person they are, what they can do what is unique about them. Highlight their strengths, their ambitions, their successes, and their visions. Knowing where they stand out is the starting point for confidence in them. A sense of direction can boost their overall perspective on life.

Take Good Care of Yourself

There's nothing wrong with having yourself pampered. You can get to places by possessing a happy spirit, a balanced body, and a content soul. Invite them to do just that. Prepare veggies for dinner, buy them supplements, and create a regular family workout regimen. Teach them how to handle disincentives, failures, and confusion. Even if trials come their way, make sure there's always hope as long as they keep an eye on themselves and don't let them crush these trials.

Accept Yourself

If you don't see it yourself, you can't make other people see your worth. Let them know they shouldn't be affected by what other people say about them. If they realize who they are and embrace themselves, they will benefit from any decision they make. Tell them what makes them happy and stick to that.

Below are A Few Tips to Help You Achieve That Goal

- Play with your child and use their name when you address them. That will make them feel unique and affectionate.

- It is encouraging when a good job is done, motivating when it's needed, and praising them for making an effort.

- When speaking with your child, always be sincere. If you just say the words and don't really pay attention, they'll know you don't mean it, and it'll lose its effectiveness.

- Reward good behavior, and discipline the child when necessary, naturally within reason.

- If something fails, let them know it's okay. They just need to make a little better preparation and try again. There's nothing wrong with occasionally failing as long as you've exhausted your best and strive to succeed in the future for betterment.

- When they talk to you, please pay attention, and engage in conversation by asking them questions. This helps develop their communication abilities and shows them how to engage in contact with others.

- Even if you disagree with something they do or believe in, let them know you value their opinions and justify why you disagree with them.

- Teaching self-confidence in your child is a vital part of their life, and they need to grow into a muscular, healthy adult. They should respect themselves and others and be proud of who they are but, at the same time, be respectful and sympathetic to others.

- Nevertheless, self-esteem should not be mistaken as vain or egotistic. There is a significant difference between raising optimistic children and brat, self-centered men. To instill the little one's self-esteem means we show them how to feel confident and content with who they are.

13.

Inspirational Activities

Montessori education integrates many activities that hone the child's skills and help him engage more in his/her interests while fostering independence and love of learning.

Here are ten inspirational activities to promote the principles of the Montessori Method:

1) Promote the Development of Body Harmony through Exercises in Precision

Let the child do what he/she is interested in. Their creativity naturally seeks to be expressed. Adults are supposed to help the child find ways to cultivate those interests and within a safe environment.

Understand that children are naturally drawn to the details. There are so many instances where parents, teachers, and other adults are surprised when a toddler or preschooler points out something that they haven't noticed.

This natural tendency to focus on details can be used to help teach children. For example, teaching handwashing can be made more interesting by giving step by step instructions. Start with where to get the materials for handwashing and close with where to put things back in their proper place.

Another method is when teaching them exercises that require fine-motor skills. For example, teaching fidgety toddlers can be made more exciting and fun by telling them to pour water without touching the water container to the glass. Make them focus on detail, and they will give their undivided attention to the activity.

Teach children as accurately as possible. Never skip or omit steps just because it is time-consuming to teach a young child. When children accurately perform activities, they can refine their motor skills.

Some of the most Montessori-recommended activities to involve children include setting up the table, serving food for meals, washing the dishes, and clearing up after meals.

2) Promote Independence in Learning by Letting Them Do Things Independently, Like Washing Their Hands After Activities

One of the core principles in Montessori is teaching children to be independent. Many parents, educators, and caregivers think that they are doing children a big favor by serving them. Serving them all their needs and doing things for them is counter-productive.

Children are naturally curious and want to try new things. Babies naturally bring items into their mouths to find out more about them.

They reach out for things, grasp, grab, and play with them; they are all ways for children to learn while developing their motor skills and mental capacities.

Just think of how a baby learns to crawl, then walk and run as he/she grows older. The parent always carries him/her everywhere or puts him/her in a baby carriage.

Therefore, it is critical to allow children to follow their nature to learn and hone skills necessary for them to grow, mature, and develop their skills, talents, and capabilities.

Parents and educators can help by not serving the child, but by providing the child opportunities to practice and to pursue their interests. Their primary responsibility is to teach children how to be independent. That includes providing opportunities for children to develop their physical motor skills. These opportunities also allow children to develop their intellectual, emotional, and social skills.

Montessori classes teach more than academics like math, language, and science. Classes also include teaching and providing children opportunities to sharpen their skills and develop their interests.

It is not surprising to see toddlers able to wash their hands and help out with cleaning up the table after meals. They also know where to get the things they need and where to put these back after use.

Patience to teach young children. It will require giving time to be with the children to guide them while they learn. But remember that while you need to let them do it themselves—you have to supervise them.

For example, adults will have to stay with the child while the child learns to pour water. Letting the child do this without supervision can lead to safety issues, like slipping and possible injuries due to spills.

3) Do Not Limit the Child Based on a Pre-conditioned Concept

One of the keys to promoting independence and the development of skills is providing opportunities for the child to practice the skills. Many parents think that their child is still too young to do something. For example, some parents think that their 3-year-old is too young to learn to wipe down a table after eating. Montessori proved that no child is too young to learn skills, especially practical life skills, like cleaning up after one's self.

Adults should show confidence in the child's ability. If a child shows a willingness to learn or to do something, let them. Just be nearby to lend assistance if needed or if something is about to go wrong.

For example, if a child wants to get a glass of water from a water dispenser, let the child do so for himself/herself. The adult should show where the child can get the cup and how to use the water dispenser. Be nearby and ready to step in if the cup is about to overflow because the child has yet to develop skill in estimating when to stop the water flow.

Adults also need to realize that children find a sense of pride and self-confidence.

4) Intervene Only When Necessary

Montessori Method is big on independence. Children work independently, but that does not mean there is no supervision present. Montessori educators are always there, observing the children.

Intervention is minimal because children are given opportunities to work things out for themselves. Teachers do not say, "That's wrong. Here's the right way to do it." Instead, children are allowed to find out for themselves where things went wrong.

The brain is naturally wired to find solutions. By letting children work independently, their brains are being trained to seek creative solutions for themselves.

This approach helps children develop creative thinking and problem-solving skills. They find their own methods of approaching problems, from perspectives that cater to their individual processes. This is more effective in teaching children than having them memorize things. This Montessori Method allows children to be active in the learning process and not mere absorbers of information.

When a teacher observes that a child made a mistake, no punishment or harsh rebuke is given. Instead, the teacher respects the child. The teacher helps the child realize what is wrong and the steps that led to the mistake. Then, the teacher allows the child to think for himself/herself on how to remedy the mistake. Activities such as those involving Knob Cylinder blocks are perfect for this.

The only time a teacher must absolutely step in is when safety is in question. The teacher must intervene in a decisive, firm manner when the child is observed doing something that might harm him/her or others.

5) Respect the Child's Autonomy

Respect for the child is utmost in the Montessori Method. Children are never forced to do something they do not want to. If a child wants to spend the morning period resting or merely observing other students, teachers allow that. There are no good results here. The child will find the school to be a bad experience. The teacher's insistent prodding will only cause the child to be more adamant in not doing any schoolwork. Forcing a child to listen to lessons won't result in any learning.

6) Include Nature

Let the child experience nature. Montessori is not about keeping children within the four walls of the classroom. It aims to develop the whole child. This includes letting the child feel oneness with nature. This is still part of providing the child opportunity to feel part of the community, including being part of the greater earth community.

Montessori also believes that being out in nature can rejuvenate the mind as well as the body. Parents are advised to bring their children outside and let them play and discover the world around them. Let the children run, crawl or roll in the grass. Let them touch the trees, leaves, the grass and the ground. This helps them develop discrimination of various textures, sizes, types of objects. There is also that refreshing feeling that only being out in nature can give and cannot be found inside the classroom.

7) Let the Child be Familiar with Social Security

Let him forms a relationship with other living creatures instead of waiting around to be given everything they want; they are given tasks that help them realize their place in society. Tasks like watering the plants and feeding pets may seem simple, but these have a considerable impact on a child. These activities help them develop compassion for other living creatures.

These teach them that there are living things that depend on them. If they do not water the plants or feed the animals, these creatures will die.

With this realization, children learn about long-term thinking. They learn to connect that what they do today is related to what happens the next day.

These activities are based on the instincts of the human soul - caring for others. A child has a nurturing instinct. Montessori knows that this child's part is just as important to cultivate as problem-solving skills or reading skills.

8) Never Speak Bad Things to and About the Child

Focus on developing and strengthening the positive aspects of a child. Ever force something that is not in the child's nature. Instead, focus on what the child is interested in and what the child shows the capacity for.

The teacher should observe the child and look for talents and strengths. Seek to include activities that allow for development. For example, a child shows a knack for visual arts. The teacher should provide more activities where the child can hone this talent. An example may be to take the child out in nature and ask the child to draw what he/she saw.

Focusing on the positives of the child's nature leaves smaller opportunities to notice the defects. This works for both the teacher and the child. When the teacher chooses to focus on the child's positive aspects, the teacher becomes less critical and more patient in dealing with the child. For the child, seeing that lessons and activities focus on his/her interests, he/she becomes more engaged, active, and focused.

Teachers, caregivers, and parents should always remember to never speak of the child in a negative way. This holds whether the child is present or not. Negative words are powerful. A single negative comment can do so much damage to a child's mental health and emotional state. It can single-handedly destroy a child's fragile sense of self.

Teach Cooperation

Cooperation can yield many prospects for the child's growth, but it requires a lot of hard work and skill. You're cooperating with the child, who is just a toddler and needs your affectionate companionship at all costs. You cannot be robust, neither you can induce horrific compulsions among them. But you must nourish the fundamentals of care and start by listening to them. You can observe their notions, and you can stay connected with their memories in a longer run. However, the question arises that what can be the potential methods of inducing cooperation in the children? Well, the answer is as follows:

Ways to be cooperative with the kids

Following are the ways to be cooperative with your kids

Taking Turns

While we are taking turns, we are boosting team management and cooperation among the toddlers. We need to understand that the baby is all growing up, and they are imitating the notions of all the elders in a respected manner. They need to understand that while growing up, the life pattern can be hazardous, and the one, who can become cooperative and compassionate, can only yearn to be successful. An example can be portrayed here to understand the thinking of the child. While they are playing blocks and or creating a puzzle, let them do their modes alternatively. It would be best if you took turns while you're building blocks for them, and then you have to see what they do in return. So, taking turns means that you have to be a team player, and you have to be cooperative with them at all costs.

Explain Your Reasons for Limits and Reasons

A controlled environment is very pertinent to reflect good progress in society. It is the only way through which success and sustainability can be achieved in the team. In this way, the house will be in order, and they will perpetually perceive management and order. Hence, this model of cooperation can be very useful for the soul and heart of the child, and you need to induce this method in all ways necessary.

Take Time to Problem Solve

You should take time to see if the kids are capable of solving the dilemmas that come in their life. Problems like the breaking of a glass, the absence of any material, and the overall loss of any prodigal thing can be termed as examples. Thus, when such dilemmas appear, the parent must ask the child many minutes and questions. Like what seems to be the problem, baby, how can the problem be solved, is there any potential solution? If so, then what is the alternative to it. When the child finds answers, and if the answers are polite and keen, then please do encourage. This encouragement will give collective clout to the children, and hence, the child will be able to yield more love for the parent.

Do Chores Together Start at an Early Age!

You need to encourage your child to do chores with you mentally. This means that if you're washing the dishes, you must allow your child to share the work burden with you. If you're washing your car, then you must bring your child into the work as well. Moreover, any burden of a work, which is being conducted and shared by you, must be allowed to be executed by your child as well. In this way, the child will learn how to cooperate with the parent and will come one step closer to the field of house-living. If you do not do it and do not allow the child to host you; properly, then you will see the negative results of their upbringing. Therefore, you must see your child get the very best of housework and do all your best in making the child look cleaner and more efficient.

Giving More Praise for Cooperative Efforts

If your child is doing something cooperatively, then do please them and give them thumbs up. Otherwise, they won't reconcile with you. The child can do a lot of work once they are given a boost and some mental encouragement. They can thaw their weaknesses and can convert them into happiness. They can see the role of their efforts progressively and can make the uttermost of the house routine. If you see others' cooperation, please do let your child learn the art of collaboration as well. Giving them more praise will clear all the mental barriers in their head about parenting, and they will come one step near you in many aspects. Thus, more recognition can lead your child to the cooperation they deserve.

Always Be Suggestive

Never be compulsive or orderly to your children. Always look to it that they have a caring parent that is suggesting them to do more and more things. If you find a mistake in them, then correct them genuinely and never let other things come in the way. Once you do bad things for the child, you will ultimately be surrounded by issues. Your child will become paranoid, and you'll make a mess of your life. Therefore, suggestions to your child will always lead to more innocence and cooperation in the child.

Give Your Child Choices While Maintaining the Rules

You are maintaining the order in your child, but at the same time, you want them to be cooperative. So, under such circumstances, it is very pertinent that you're suggestive of your child's actions and let the child be on the same path with you. For instance, before bed, if you want your child to follow the rules, ask them politely if they have brushed their teeth, and are their diapers clean. These cute and innocent questions will liberate the child from tension, and they will cooperate more.

Explain Them the Situations in a Calm Manner

Explain to them the reasons why low expectations come in the way. And do not yell at them while you're doing so. If, by chance, they cannot clear any exam, then it isn't your obligation to defame them. Just be a kind parent and let them understand the possibilities of life in an affectionate manner. Try to suggest more cooperative tactics that will enable them to yearn enjoyment. So, the explanation of challenging situations in an easy way will make your child more cooperative and substantial.

Play Games with Them

Games like cricket and football are very significant to boost creativity and subjectivity in the kids. If you hold a bat and hit your child's ball, the child will learn cooperation by all means necessary. Even if you're playing the game of football with them and running alongside them and telling them how to kick, then you are cooperative, and the child will be more productive to your advice and learning. Therefore, play as much of the games you want to play with them, and in the end, you'll end up being very affectionate with them. Splendid methods make the child know the cooperation platform and feel proud if you're doing so.

Always Ask Permission Before Joining

Always ask your child permissions if you're about to join them and see what the child can do. If your child is playing the match of cricket and watching them, try your best not to disturb them; if you're washing the dishes and the child is watching movies, ask their permission to join them. These examples assert your cooperative and affectionate behavior with the child and, eventually, lead the child to a better end. But if you are arrogant and stubborn enough to scold them vociferously, then you must not expect any kind of cooperation from the child. Because the child will be very stubborn for you, and they won't learn the art of collaboration.

Sharing Is Caring

If you're a busy guy and have a strict schedule on your time, try your best to comply with your child. Understandably, the child will not get your routine, and with innocent questions and a jolly mood, everybody can calm down. For instance, the child can get to the bottom of your routine, and you're having a tough time dealing with them so, in such a circumstance, you must adhere to all the disciplinary steps that can navigate obedience in your child and hence, you need to share things with him, to achieve cooperation from their side. Hence, they will care for you if you share your routine with them.

So, with such ways and measures, the term cooperation can be easily put forward to the students and children.

14.

Self-discovering

The Montessori Method of teaching has a unique aspect in it that is known as self-discovering. It is an indulging process due to which an individual can manifest new things in themself. These things are not explained before to the individuals, and by the passage of time, they tend to discover something in them as a result of active effort and brainstorming. With its specialized gadget of a broad curriculum, the Montessori method allows individuals to find self-discovery modes in them. The following are some of the children's tactics and frameworks while they are self-discovering themselves.

Through the years, discovery through Montessori has proven to be an excellent and effective way for children to learn. As the children go through the Montessori classroom's different learning areas, they know the concepts and skills they need to enrich their education. As you watch any child go into such a classroom, you will marvel at how they can learn without much help from their teachers.

Decision-Making: Allowing Children to Make Their Own Choices

Decision making and a child's choice are integral elements of the Montessori method. As the parent, you're aware that you act as a guide, merely a way-shower and support system for your child's journey. Allowing your child to choose their course of action and activity engagement opens up new pathways for individual skills, talents, and gifts to shine through. If the choice is taken away and they are made to conform to a rigid structure and 'one way' way of doing things, they are less likely to step fully into their self-expression and special personal qualities. Everyone is unique, and Montessori aims to bring this to the forefront.

Visual Learning

Visual learning is learning through visual representations, such as images, written material, video, or whiteboards. Visual learning involves taking in a range of sensory information through the sense of sight.

Auditory or Musical Learning

Auditory learning is learning through sound. Auditory learners process information and concepts best when heard or listened to. They are also the types of learners who learn best using rhythm or melody; thus, they are also known as musical learners. For instance, musicians learn best by listening to a specific musical piece. Then they try playing the same amount from memory. These learners may also learn more effectively when there's music playing on the background or when they're whistling, humming, toe-tapping, and doing some musical or rhythmic action while learning.

Kinesthetic Learning

Kinesthetic learners understand and process information best when actively engaged in it, such as through touch or using their bodies and movement to acquire knowledge. These learners love interacting with the world around them since it is how they learn. They are scientific, and they enjoy hands-on learning, which is perfect because Montessori is all about hands-on activities.

Linguistic Learning

Linguistic learners are the ones that learn best when they're able to use linguistic skills such as speaking, listening, writing, and reading. It's even better when they're able to learn through a combination of these different skills and methods.

Naturalist Learning

Naturalist learners are the ones that learn best by experience and working with nature. When you think about naturalist learners, an image of a scientist may come to your mind. This would be entirely accurate because a lot of scientists are naturalist learners. They love to observe the world around them; they love experiencing their world, and they learn more effectively through experimentation.

Teach Compassion

Teaching compassion through activities and exercises which involve love and respect for animals and ecosystems is a great and effective way to enhance your child's empathic nature. Many children are already naturally empathic - it is the world and some of the societal practices and structures in play that make them less so. We are born with a natural sensitivity and compassion towards sentient creatures, and this is often displayed through many acts of kindness shown by the children. Feeling genuine sadness and empathy towards animals, questioning the process of eating them, and feeling plants and other nature on a deep level are all common occurrences. The Montessori framework is ideal for developing this natural compassion and connecting to a child's empathic nature.

Practicing Kindness

Practicing and acknowledging kindness in the classroom or environment you have created for learning and activity is another way to develop empathy. This can be done by offering praise, where appropriate, and words of support and encouragement, such as 'that was nice of you,' 'that was very thoughtful and considerate,' or 'it was very kind of you to do this.' Remember, you are a guide for your child or children, so supporting efforts through verbal recognition will further increase the kindness and compassion they are already exhibiting. Try and not to overdo it, though, as too much attention to the natural kind and empathic displays can have the opposite effect, bringing focus to your child's pride and praise instead of the acts they are engaging in.

Being Respectful

It is very accurate to suggest that learning, by example, is one of the most effective ways to learn. Showing respect and treating your child as a young adult, or an equal is possibly one of the most powerful ways to be an example of empathy. Showing respect to objects, learning material, things in your environment, and other humans, plants, and animals will directly influence your child or children.

Self-Care

When students or toddlers come into the Montessori School, they are taught to self-care themselves. They are trained to learn the most favorable aspects of themselves, and by doing so, they care for themselves. Dynamically, the children understand that what is meant by self-respect, self-mannerism, and self-dignity is that they would not shout loud or make obscene gestures. Moreover, the toddlers are given independent environments, where they can grow sustainably. The toddlers can get a huge amount of understanding for themselves, and thus, for more extended means, the toddlers can get to care themselves profusely. Thus, the much-anticipated aspect of love is self-care, and self-discovering helps the infants grow more effectively.

Caring for the Environment

The toddlers are taught to care for the enviromnent. Although they are very young and need to be careful while they chose the right environment to stay, the Montessori School regards the ideal features for their children. In the initial months of school, the toddlers are taught how to clean the environment by showing them the cleaning art. They are given some woolen cloths so that the children can easily tide the nearby dirt with full zeal. Hence, the caring of the environment is a chief aspect of self-discovering for the toddlers, and it is taught nowhere but by the Montessori School.

Development of Motor Skills

Motor skills are essential for a child to come across. These skills give the horary values of a good citizen and a punctual human being. These skills further enhance the aptitude of young schoolers and give them a reason to succeed in life. These skills include walking, climbing, running, and jumping. Children tend to discover their athleticism through these skills, and in the future, they get more successful while doing it. Thus, the development of motor skills is yet another aspect of self-discovery, and it is given by the Montessori School in all the possible manners holistically.

Language Learning

Language learning is yet another exciting art that needs to be accumulated by the students at all rates possible. This is a conversational approach that needs to be given to all the toddlers in the initial phase of their lifelines. They are taught how to converse on pictures. They are trained to name the objects; the students' singing is related to the students' cognition. Thus, numerically, people can discuss the importance of self-discovering. The mode of self-discovering is accelerated when language learning is more acceptable. Therefore, the Montessori School shares its pride in fostering more and more productive avenues for the classmates.

Social Skills

The Montessori School teaches social skills to infants about how they need to behave with the colored babies and how to be compatible with people in various ways. Social skills give the students more enhanced capabilities to reach more progress in their mental skills and other developmental skills. From a young age, they learn the edifices of tolerance, mutual acceptability, and sympathy. In social skills, the toddlers and infants are taught how to shake hands and how to be more convincing for others to be with them.

Language Development Activities

Object and Sound Comparison: From around your home, gather a selection of items that your child is very familiar with and can name. These can either be household items or play toys. Sandpaper Letters: The letter blocks are easy to make if you would not invest in a premade set. Trace and cut out the entire alphabet on pieces of sandpaper. Each letter should be a few inches in height. Ensure that the script you use is consistent throughout and stick to either upper- or lower-case letters. Once you have the letters cut out, adhere them to small boards of a contrasting color. Most Montessori schools prefer to start with lower-case cursive.

Movable Alphabet Word Formation: While it is possible to use a simple set of refrigerator magnets for this activity, it is advised that you either purchase or make a particular set of the moveable alphabet, with one color designated for consonants and the other for vowels. The color differentiation helps the child to recognize the different roles of the letters.

Chalk Letter Writing: Sometimes, Montessori activities are so simple that they seem almost too obvious. When you encounter these activities, take a moment to think about what other ways your child's educational experience can be enriched by participation.

Phonetic SoundBox: This is an activity using the phonetic soundbox aimed toward the older child that is getting closer to independent reading. Find several items from around your home that have short spellings with sounds that can be easily decoded. For example, pen, tag, cup, dot, etc.

Mathematical Development Activities

Sandpaper Numbers: Nearly identical in presentation to the sandpaper letters used above, sandpaper numbers will teach your child how to write numbers and reinforce each visual representation's name correctly. The numbers used should be zero to nine; however, zero should not be introduced until the child has had an opportunity to learn and understand none. This seems pretty basic, though, to a young child associating order and quantity to a visual number, it can be challenging to grasp nothingness.

Spindle Box: For this activity, you need a spindle box and a complete set of spindles. This is also one of those pieces of equipment that can easily be created if you do not wish to purchase one. All you need is a long box, with enough dividers to separate the box into compartments numbered zero through nine. You will also need enough small rods for the child to place the appropriate number into each slot.

Number Rods: Number rods are excellent for introducing a variety of mathematical concepts and are an excellent investment for your Montessori home school as you will have continued use of this product for at least a couple of years. A good number rod set will include instructions for several activities, the most basic of which is a simple ordering exercise that will help introduce the rods' concept to your child.

CPSIA information can be obtained
at www.ICGtesting.com
Printed in the USA
BVHW062003250321
603411BV00002B/159